LONG TERM CARE MONITORING TOOLS
FOR
RESIDENT MEAL TIME AND DINING EXPERIENCE
AND
KITCHEN AND FOOD SERVICE

authorHOUSE®

AuthorHouse™
1663 Liberty Drive
Bloomington, IN 47403
www.authorhouse.com
Phone: 1-800-839-8640

Published by AuthorHouse 6/13/2012

ISBN: 978-1-4685-8541-4 (e)
ISBN: 978-1-4685-8542-1 (sc)

Library of Congress Control Number: 2012910658

LONG TERM CARE MONITORING TOOLS
FOR
RESIDENT MEAL TIME AND DINING EXPERIENCE
AND
KITCHEN AND FOOD SERVICE

Nora Wellington

This book with the accompanying monitoring tools for the related Federal Regulations, and F-tags is designed to help staff monitor for survey preparedness and for maintaining compliance. It is not the intention of the author that this book be used as the only source for survey preparation, or for compliance with the related F-tags.

The author encourages facility staff to utilize this book in addition to the Federal long term care regulations and other State regulatory materials. This book should not be a substitute for the Federal Long Term Care Regulations and Interpretive Guidelines or the State Long Term Care Regulations.

Arrangements can be made for quantity discounts. For more information, please contact:

N Wellington Associates LLC
2903 Radius Road
Wheaton, MD 20902

Telephone: (301) 933-9246
Email: nora_w@nwellingtonassociates.com
Website: www.nwellingtonassociates.com

Table of Contents

Acknowledgments

This is to say special thanks to my friends and colleagues, and also to other long term care professionals and facility administrators who have purchased my first book, "The Fundamentals of Quality for Long Term Care Part 1". I appreciate the positive feedback I received from my colleagues. To the other facility administrators, I hope that you and your staff also found the book useful and beneficial. I also welcome feedback from you.

To my sister, Alicia Creighton-Allen, who co-authored the first book with me, thank you. It was a great experience working with you on the project.

To my good friend and colleague, who will remain nameless for now; and his staff, who took the time to review and edited this book, Long Term Care Monitoring Tools, I thank you. I appreciate you reviewing the book for accuracy of content and quality. I appreciate your continuous support. I also thank my sister Gloria Allen who did the initial editing of the manuscript. I appreciate you giving of your time.

To my husband Dudley, thank you your love and support. To my sons, Dudley II and Neal thank you very much also for your love and continuous support; I am very grateful. I also give special thanks to Neal for designing the cover of the book Long Term Care Monitoring Tools. When I explained what I wanted the cover to look like, you did a very good job transferring my thoughts to the cover. Thank you for coming up with this beautiful cover that portrays the essence of the book.

I want to use this opportunity to honor the Food Service staff, the Dietitians, the Certified Nursing Assistants, Feeding Assistants, Charge Nurses, and all staffs who routinely take on the responsibility for making sure the residents have good nutritious meals and satisfying meal time experiences in their Homes (the long term care facilities). The reality is that, these staff more often than not hear the phrase "I don't like this food, please give me something else". So these staffs have to stay on top of the residents' food preferences, and choices. Thank you for your contribution to making sure the residents enjoy their meals.

About the Author

Nora J. Wellington, MBA, NHA, is a long term care consultant, CEO / Founder of N Wellington Associates LLC (www.nwellingtonassociates.com) , and co- author of The Fundamentals of Quality for Long Term Care Part 1. Wellington has more than twenty-five years of long term care (LTC) experience, including nineteen years as a nursing home administrator who operated and managed skilled nursing facilities and nursing facilities.

Wellington was fortunate to be hired fifteen years ago to help a hospital open a brand new subacute/skilled nursing unit. She worked with the director of nursing, and the hospital's project director to develop the required clinical and administrative policies and procedures to present to the District of Columbia Department of Health for approval.

She developed educational in-services on long term care regulations, survey protocol and the importance of regulatory compliance for the in-coming administrative and clinical staff and for physicians. She led the staff through the initial Medicare and Medicaid certification survey to operate the facility. Wellington also prepared the staff and led them through the joint commission long term care certification survey.

Wellington loved being a hands-on administrator during her nineteen years as administrator at her facilities, because it gave her the opportunity to be close to the staff while obtaining an in-depth experience of operational issues. She has designed several monitoring tools for use internally in the facilities that she has served as administrator. Wellington has a passion for teaching and training staff at all levels. She has also designed training workshops on topics such as "Effective Communication Skills with Focus on Assertiveness", "Customer Service Effectiveness", and "Team Building" for small size organizations.

Wellington graduated with BA in Business Administration from Howard University, and an MBA from George Washington University, both in Washington, DC. She also attended the University of Maryland University College (UMUC) to do her course work in Gerontology, Ageing & Disability, and Long Term Care Administration. Because of her desire to continue to teach as well as to learn, Wellington took the professional business coaching training.

In addition to her professional business career, Wellington serves her community as chairman of her church board (Sr. Warden of the Vestry) of her Episcopal church in Maryland. To further her outreach work, she is developing workshops on "healthcare delivery to seniors" within her local faith communities. She also is a member of the American College of Health Care Administrators, a VIP member of the National Association of Professional Women, and member of GROWS – Grass Roots Organization for the Well-being of Seniors.

Introduction

The Centers for Medicare and Medicaid Services (CMS) expect all Skilled Nursing Facilities (SNFs) and Nursing Facilities (NFs) to routinely stay in substantial compliance of the Federal Long Term Care Regulations 42 CFR §483.5 – §483.75. Attaining, maintaining and sustaining this goal on an ongoing consistent basis does take a lot of hard work, commitment and dedicated staff time for regular ongoing monitoring of quality of care, quality of life, and safety of the environment that facilities provide for the residents and the families they serve.

It is the practice for Administrators to make available for staffs, copies of the Federal long term care regulations, State long term care regulations, State Operations Manual, Survey and Enforcement Protocol and other long term care manuals. Keeping abreast of all regulations, new information and quality initiatives sometimes present a challenge to some facilities. Staff assimilating the breadth of all the regulations is itself not an easy task; but the importance of staffs knowing those parts of the regulations that pertain to their disciplines cannot be over-emphasized.

Having an *easy-to-read and easy-to-follow* book and monitoring tools focusing on select disciplines and/or departments will assist staffs increase their knowledgebase of these regulations. CMS has established ongoing routine monitoring as one of their expectations for SNFs and NFs. We know that facilities do establish plans for routine monitoring, however those plans get held back sometimes by unexpected realities such as staff call-ins, or incidences that have to be attended to. But routine monitoring none the less, should not be put on hold.

The purpose of this book is to assist Administrators, Directors of Nursing, Directors of Quality Assurance/Quality Improvement, Directors / Coordinators of Staff Development **help the facility staff to:**

- Get to know those F-tags that are relevant to Residents Meal Time & Dining Experience, and Kitchen & Food Service.

- Make the F-tags and the Regulations for Residents Meal Time & Dining Experience and Kitchen & Food Service, the foundation while they are providing care.

- Monitor, monitor, and then monitor.

- Understand important relevant definitions, and the Survey and Enforcement Protocol, including enforcement remedies.

To administrators and staff: we all know that an increase in one's knowledgebase and one's comfort level of the regulations and the F-tags makes preparing for survey a little easier; and keeping abreast of the continuous quality initiatives from CMS and other stakeholders also becomes a little less burdensome. These *easy-to-read Resident Meal Time and Dining Experience, and Kitchen and Food Service Monitoring Tools* with the question format and the Synopsis of the Survey and Enforcement Protocol will help staff with survey preparation and ongoing quality of care and quality of life monitoring.

Concerning the new Quality Indicator Survey (QIS) methodology, CMS has transitioned some States survey agencies to the QIS format, but others are still being surveyed by the Traditional Survey methodology. The QIS implementation schedule has been set with a target date for all facilities in the nation to become QIS by 2015. If your facility is not yet QIS do not worry, CMS and your State will let you know when you are scheduled to transition to QIS; and your staff will be trained. QIS methodology is a computer assisted methodology which was introduced to improve the consistency and accuracy of quality of care and quality of life problem identification by surveyors. Part 1 of this book gives a brief description of the survey process.

CMS continues to make this very important point that **"the Federal Long Term Care Regulations remain the same; they have not changed"**. So the introduction of the QIS does not affect the regulations or the Survey and Enforcement remedies.

When staffs get into the habit of routine weekly ongoing monitoring this will generally impact in a positive way the facility's survey preparedness and readiness. All SNFs and NFs are required to be in compliance with the *42 CFR, Part 483, Subpart B* in order to receive and continue to receive payment under the Medicare and Medicaid programs. The survey process is designed to show facilities areas of non compliance with the long term care requirements. In this book I have combined the brief synopsis of the survey and enforcement protocol with the monitoring tools to help staff make the connection of the whole process in a real way, in order to improve compliance with the regulations and avoid remedies levied by CMS.

This book is divided into three parts as outlined below.

- **Part I** contains **important Definitions, Survey Protocol and Process from the State Operations Manual**. These are select definitions, and the survey process that every staff should know and become familiar with.

- **Part II** contains **Monitoring Tools for both Resident Meal Time & Dining Experience and Kitchen & Food Service.**

- **Part III** contains brief Synopsis of the **Enforcement Protocol** with a listing of **Remedies for non compliance of the Federal Regulations**

This book is based on the current Federal Long Term Care Regulations and the Survey and Enforcement Protocol.

PART I

STATE OPERATIONS MANUAL APPENDIX P

BRIEF SYNOPSIS

DEFINITIONS

&

SURVEY PROCESS

PART I

State Operations Manual Appendix P

Synopsis of Portions of the State Operations Manual:

Survey Protocol for Long Term Care Facilities, Appendix P

Identifying Different Types of Survey

The Standard Survey for both Traditional Survey and Quality Indicator Survey (QIS) is defined in Appendix P, as "resident-centered, outcome-oriented inspections that rely on a case-mix stratified sample of residents to gather information about the facility's compliance with participation requirements". Results of a survey may include actual and potential negative outcomes, as well as failure of a facility to help residents achieve their highest practicable level of well-being.

A standard survey for a long term care facility assesses:

- Compliance with residents' rights and quality of life requirements as outlined in the regulations;

- The accuracy of residents' comprehensive assessments and the adequacy of care plans, the timeliness of care plans including revisions as needed, based on these assessments;

- The quality of care and services provided to the residents, as measured by indicators of medical, nursing, rehabilitative care and drug therapy, dietary and nutrition services, activities and social participation, sanitation and infection control; and

- The effectiveness of the physical environment to empower residents, accommodate resident needs, and maintain resident safety, and also whether requested room variances, if any, meet the health, safety, and quality of life needs for the affected residents.

The standard survey measures how well a skilled nursing facility and a nursing facility maintain compliance with the regulations relative to Quality of Life, Quality of Care, and Life Safety of the residents. It must also be noted that these long term care regulations are the minimum standards required for facilities, so facilities need to set a goal of not only meeting these standards but also of exceeding these standards.

Additional Survey Types for Traditional Survey Facilities

In addition to the Standard Survey, listed below are **additional survey types** that all staff must also know.

Another type of survey is an **Extended Survey. An extended survey** is conducted if the survey team determines that substandard quality of care exist during the standard survey. If it is determined by the surveyors that the facility has provided substandard quality of care, in violation of 42 CFR 483.13, Resident Behavior and Facility Practices; 42 CFR 483.15, Quality of Life; and /or 42 CFR 483.25 Quality of Care, the surveyors will conduct an extended survey **within 14 days** after completion of the standard survey.

If a resident or a family member files a complaint with the State Survey Agency, the surveyors will pay a visit to your facility in response to the complaint. They will perform what is called an **Abbreviated Standard Survey** that focuses on a particular task. The particular task will focus on the issues and concerns of the complaint(s) received. Also if there is a change of ownership, or a change in management, or a change in director of nursing at a facility, surveyors may conduct an abbreviated standard survey at that facility.

While surveyors are performing an abbreviated survey, if the surveyors find troubling **substandard quality of care issue(s),** they will perform a **Partial Extended Survey.** The surveyors will also conduct the partial extended survey after a substandard quality of care is determined during a revisit, even though substandard quality of care was not previously identified during the original standard survey.

A **Post-Survey Revisit or Follow-Up** is an onsite visit or survey intended to verify correction of deficiencies cited in the prior survey. The surveyors will review the plan of correction submitted by the facility, with the goal of assessing whether the deficiencies cited have been corrected as outlined in the plan of correction.

Initial Certification Survey for a Skilled Nursing Facility (SNF) and/or Nursing Facility (NF) is defined as that survey which incorporates both a Traditional Standard Survey and Extended Survey. At this initial survey the surveyors focus on both the residents and the structural requirements that relate to qualification standards and residents notification, whether or not problems are identified during the information gathering tasks. They also focus on policies and procedures. The surveyors will gather information to verify compliance on every tag number.

The Different Types of Survey for the Quality Indicator Survey Version

The Quality Indicator Survey (QIS) process is currently being used only to survey facilities in states where CMS has approved the utilization of QIS. CMS has established its implementation timeline and the surveyors follow the timeline as established. The implementation process involves training of surveyors, training of the facilities within that State, and the readiness by the states for the transition from Traditional Survey to the Quality Indicator Survey.

The QIS Standard Survey - CMS describes QIS as a two-staged process used by surveyors to systematically review specific nursing home requirements and objectively investigate any regulatory areas that are triggered. Stage I is called the information gathering stage which provides for an initial review of large samples of residents. It also involves observation by surveyors of staff and residents, and also observation of the environment. The sampling involves not only record review but it also involves interview of the residents, their families, and also staff interviews. This stage incorporates the utilization of an onsite automation process to determine areas that are triggered for care investigation. Stage II allows surveyors to use investigative protocols to systematically review triggered care areas, complete mandatory facility-level tasks, and triggered facility-level tasks such as abuse prevention, environment, nursing services, sufficient staffing, personal funds, and admission, transfer and discharge.

The QIS Extended Survey – when the survey team is conducting a QIS standard survey and they have determined that there is substandard quality of care, they will conduct QIS extended survey. The purpose of the QIS extended survey is to gather further information concerning the facility's operations including nursing services, medical services and administration. The surveyors will evaluate systemic issues with the facility's provision of services including management that may have contributed to the non-compliance and sub-standard quality of care. The areas of focus will be *42 CFR 483.13*, Resident Behavior and Facility Practices, *42 CFR 483.15*, Quality of Life, and *42 CFR 483.25*, Quality of Care.

Survey and Enforcement Process for Skilled Nursing Facilities and Nursing Facilities (Rev. 63, Effective 09-10-10, Implemented 09-10-10)

CMS through the State Operations Manual has outlined the following expectations for Skilled Nursing Facilities (SNFs) and Nursing Facilities (NFs). The expectations are as follows:

- The first expectation is that Providers must remain in substantial compliance with Medicare/Medicaid program. The regulation emphasizes the need for continued, rather than cyclical compliance.[1]

- The second expectation is that all deficiencies will be addressed promptly. The standard for program participation mandated by the regulation is substantial compliance.[2]

- The third expectation is that residents will receive the care and services they need to meet highest practicable level of functioning.[3]

As a long term care professional or a staff that cares for our elderly seniors, are you familiar with your profession's terminologies? I am listing below some important terminologies with the corresponding definitions. All staffs, including nurse managers, charge nurses, medication nurses, certified nursing assistants, feeding assistants, directors of nursing, social workers, activities professional, food service workers, food service directors, dietitians, and administrators must know these long term care terminologies.

Definitions of Selected Terms as defined by CMS in Chapter 7 of the State Operations Manual:

Abuse – is defined as the willful infliction of injury, unreasonable confinement, intimidation, or punishment with resulting physical harm, pain, or mental anguish. (*42 CFR 488.301*)

CMS – is the Centers for Medicare & Medicaid Services (formerly known as HCFA)

Deficiency – is defined as a skilled nursing facility's or nursing facility's failure to meet a participation requirement specified in the Act or in 42 CFR Part 483 Subpart B. (*42 CFR 488.301*)

Educational program – is defined as programs that include any subject pertaining to the long term care participation requirements, the survey process, or the enforcement process.

Enforcement action – is defined as the process of imposing one or more of the following remedies: termination of a provider agreement; denial of participation; denial of payment for new admissions; denial of payment for all residents; temporary manager; civil money penalty; State monitoring; directed plan of correction; directed in-service training; transfer of residents; closure of the facility and transfer of residents; or other CMS approved alternative State remedies.

Expanded survey – is defined as an increase beyond the core tasks of a standard survey. When surveyors suspect substandard quality of care they should expand the survey to determine if substandard quality of care does exist.

Extended survey – is defined as a survey that evaluates additional participation requirements subsequent to finding substandard quality of care during standard survey.

Immediate jeopardy – is defined as a situation in which the facility's noncompliance with one or more requirement of participation has caused, or is likely to cause, serious injury, harm, impairment, or death to a resident. (*42 CFR 488.301*)

Misappropriation of resident property – is defined as the deliberate misplacement, exploitation, or wrongful, temporary or permanent use of a resident's belongings or money without the resident's consent.

Neglect – is defined as failure to provide goods and services necessary to avoid physical harm, mental anguish, or mental illness. (*42 CFR 488.301*)

Noncompliance – is defined as any deficiency that causes a facility not to be in substantial compliance. (*42 CFR 488.301*)

Nursing facility – is defined as a Medicaid nursing facility.

Per instance civil money penalty – is defined as a civil money penalty imposed for each instance of facility noncompliance.

Skilled nursing facility – is defined as a Medicare-certified nursing facility that has a Medicare provider agreement.

Standard survey – is defined as a periodic, resident-centered inspection that gathers information about the quality of service furnished in a facility to determine compliance with the requirements of participation.

Substandard quality of care – is defined as one or more deficiencies related to participation requirements under *42 CFR 483.13*, resident behavior and facility practices, *42 CFR 483.15*, quality of life, or *42 CFR 483.25*, quality of care, that constitute either immediate jeopardy to resident health or safety (level J, K, or L); a pattern of or widespread actual harm that is not immediate jeopardy (level H or I); or a widespread potential for more than minimal harm, but less than immediate jeopardy, with no actual harm (level F). (*42 CFR 499.301*)

Substantial compliance – is defined as a level of compliance with the requirements of participation mandated by CMS such that any identified deficiencies pose no greater risk to resident health or safety than the potential for causing minimal harm. Substantial compliance constitutes compliance with participation requirements, (*42 CFR 488.301*). In terms of a certification survey, Substantial compliance also means that a facility has a successful survey.

Survey Protocol and Survey Process
Traditional Survey

Skilled Nursing Facilities (SNF) and Nursing Facilities (NF) undergo standard surveys annually, as part of certification process for continued participation in the Medicare and Medicaid programs. In this section a brief summary of the survey process for a Traditional Survey will be presented. The annual certification survey is usually performed by a survey team which comprises a Team Coordinator/Leader, and surveyors with different clinical skills. The survey team usually is staff of the State Survey Agency, and they perform the survey function on behalf of the Federal Government if the facility is a Medicare/Medicaid Facility. Please note that the phrase "survey team" and the word "surveyors" may be used interchangeably in this book.

Federal Surveyors periodically will team up with the State Surveyors to perform standard certification surveys at facilities. Federal surveyors periodically may also conduct what is called "look back". The "look back" is when Federal Surveyors conduct a survey at a facility approximately three or four weeks after the state surveyors finish their survey.

Whether the State surveyors perform surveys at the facilities by themselves or whether they team up with the Federal surveyors, I am outlining below a summary of the survey process and tasks performed by the survey team.

1. **Pre-survey preparation usually called Offsite Survey Preparation.** The survey team coordinator or team leader and survey team will:
   - Review the previous survey deficiency results and plan of correction of the facility they plan to survey.
   - Review the facility's complaint surveys and any current complaint not yet addressed.
   - Talk to the Ombudsman to find out if there have been complaints about the facility.
   - Identify areas of concerns.

2. **Entrance Conference** - the team coordinator will meet with the Administrator, and the Director of Nursing, and introduce the team. The team coordinator will give the administrator a two page list of information/documents needed by the survey team. The information/documents requested are listed in #3 through #8 below.

3. After the **introduction,** the other members of the team will tour the facility as part of the **initial tour** of the facility. The team coordinator soon thereafter will:
   - Ask the administrator for the actual work schedule of the licensed practical nursing and registered nursing staff for the current period.
   - Give the administrator his/her copy of the CASPER 3 & CASPER 4 (due to the new MDS 3.0, the Quality Measure/Quality Indicator (QM/QI) cannot be used until further notice).

- Ask the administrator if there any new programs that have been implemented since the facility's last survey.
- Ask the administrator if the facility utilizes paid feeding assistants – if the facility does, the administrator will be asked to provide information as to when and where the feeding assistants received their training. If the paid feeding assistants went through a State approved program. Paid feeding assistants also must work under the supervision of a licensed practical nurse (LPN) or a registered nurse (RN)
- Ask the administrator about the facility's Quality Assurance (Q.A.) Committee and more importantly, with whom should the survey team discuss Q.A. issues.

4. The information/documents listed below must be provided by the administrator **within one hour** of the end of the entrance conference.
   - List of key personnel of the facility.
   - The information provided to residents regarding their rights.
   - Meal time, dining location(s), and copies of menus.
   - Medication pass times
   - List of new admissions within the past month, and list of discharges within the past three months with the discharge destination.
   - Copy of the facility's layout.
   - Copy of the facility's admission's contract.
   - Copy of the facility's policies and procedures on "prevention of abuse".
   - Evidence that the facility monitors incidents and accidents.
   - Names of residents aged 55 and younger.
   - Names of residents who communicate with non-oral communication devices, sign language, or who speak different language as dominant language.

5. This document listed below must be provided by the Director of Nursing before the end of **the initial tour.**
   - The Director of Nursing will make available to the team coordinator a completed **Roster/Sample Matrix (Form CMS-802).** This is the total census in a matrix format, including residents on "bed-hold". This is vital information that the survey team needs as part of the sample selection process.

6. The following documents must be provided by the administrator **within 24 hours of the Entrance Conference.**
   - A completed Long Term Care Facility Application for Medicare and Medicaid Form CMS-671
   - A resident Census and Conditions of Residents Form CMS-672
   - A list of Medicare residents who requested Demand Bills within the last 6 months.

7. The administrator will go through a **Question and Answer session** with the Team Coordinator. Such questions asked of the administrator are:
   - Is there any room in the facility that does not meet requirement for which the facility has been granted variance?
   - Are there any rooms in the facility occupied by more than four residents?
   - Is there at least one window to the outside in each room?
   - Are there any bedrooms that are not above ground level?
   - Do all bedrooms have access to an exit corridor?
   - What are the facility's procedures if there is a loss of normal water supply?

8. The team coordinator will ask the administrator to **post signs announcing that a survey** is being performed at the facility. These signs should be posted in high visibility areas such as the lobby of the facility.

9. The team coordinator will also contact the president of the Resident Council, to introduce him or herself, and to also let the president of the resident council know that a survey is being performed.

10. The team coordinator or designee will schedule a private or group interview with the resident council.

11. It must be noted that there are times when surveyors will start the survey on an evening or on Saturday or Sunday. Whenever this happens the survey team coordinator will ask for the person in charge of the facility at that time, and also ask that the administrator be contacted and informed to let him/her know that the survey has begun. The team coordinator will make adjustments as to when certain documents are needed. Please note that the survey continues with the staff on duty at that time.

The Initial Tour

The initial tour by the survey team is the opportunity for the surveyors to gather information about the **concerns that the team had preselected** during the offsite preparation stage. It also is the opportunity for the surveyors to get an impression of the environment, the kitchen and food service department. The team coordinator will designate each team member to tour individually a different area of the facility.

It is always advisable for the facility Director of Nursing to have a knowledgeable facility staff member who is familiar with the residents on the unit, go around with the assigned survey team member, so the staff can answer questions posed by the survey team member. The survey team members will document their findings on these focal areas:

- Concerns about the residents
- Concerns about the general environment
- Concerns about the facility kitchen or Food service

Concerns about the Residents

During the initial tour the survey team members will identify new concerns based on their observations or from information obtained from staff. The areas that the survey members will briefly look at include Quality of Life, Resident Behavior / Facility Practices, and Quality of Care.

For Quality of Life the surveyors will observe or ask questions about:
- Resident grooming and dress – do residents have food stains on their clothing?
- Resident privacy – does staff maintain residents' privacy?
- Resident dignity – does staff call residents by name?
- Courtesy to resident – how does staff talk to residents?
- Scheduled recreational activities taking place, or not taking place

For Resident Behavior and Facility Practices the surveyors will observe or ask questions about:
- Resident behaviors such as crying, disrobing, rocking, pacing
- Resident behavior such as agitation
- Staff interaction with residents – how well does staff interact with residents?
- The manner in which the resident behaviors are being addressed by staff, including staff's response time to meeting residents' needs
- How long the call bell rings before it is answered – promptly or delay in responding?

For Quality of Care issues the surveyors will observe or ask questions about:
- Skin condition – excessive dryness, or wetness
- Skin tears or bruising, etc.
- Evidence of whether hydration is addressed, is there water at bedside for resident; other risk factors for dehydration – color of urine in tubing or collection bag, strong urine odor, etc.
- Positioning of residents sitting in wheelchairs – how well are residents positioned?
- Use of physical restraints – how many residents have physical restraint?
- Presence or prevalence of infections, e.g. MRSA, VRE, C-Diff, UTI, etc.
- Pressure sores, or old scars from pressure sores

- Dietary issues e.g. significant weight loss
- Feeding tubes and/or improper positioning of resident while feeding is infusing
- Ventilators, oxygen, and intravenous therapies – observation of nurses providing care

Concerns about the General Environment

The surveyors will observe or will ask questions of the staff about:
- How safe does the environment look for the residents - Are there equipments left unattended in the hallway?
- Functional and clean equipments on the units.
- Maintenance of equipment – preventive maintenance program.
- Availability of assistive devices for residents' use.
- The important infection control practices – hand washing, usage of gloves.
- Residents on isolation – isolation protocol followed by staff and visitors?

Concerns about the Kitchen

The surveyors will observe or ask questions of the food service staff about:
- Sanitation practices of the food service staff.
- The cleanliness of the kitchen.
- The storing, preparing, distributing and serving of food in accordance with regulations.
- Leaving food on the counter tops and steam tables – potential for hazardous situation.
- Thawing of food
- Cleanliness of attire of food service staff – Are staffs wearing uniforms or are they wearing street clothes?
- Attire of head coverings of food staff – hairnets, etc.

Phase 2 of the Survey

After the Offsite Preparation, the Entrance Conference, and the Initial Tour, the survey team would have collected enough information to identify the areas of concern they want to look at and to also complete the selection of the remainder of the sample of residents for the survey.

Concerns selection at this point of the survey is based on the following: (1) offsite concerns and initial tour concerns that have not been reviewed; (2) new concerns during the initial tour that have not yet been investigated; (3) concerns that may have been identified as a result of other care concerns; (4) and current concerns for which information gathered may be inconclusive.

The completion of the resident sampling involves what is called in the statutes "case mix stratified" sample. CMS requires that the stratification includes residents who are interviewable and residents who are non-interviewable, and also should include residents who require heavy care as well as residents who require light care. Also the team will select residents who represent one or more of the areas of concerns identified. Because hydration is such an important care issue, one or more residents will be selected in the sampling that has risk factor for dehydration.

Special factors also come into play in the sampling selection process based on the case-mix stratification process. Such special factors include selecting residents who:
- Are newly admitted within 14 days of the start of the survey
- Have conditions that put them at risk for neglect or abuse, such as residents with dementia, or who have some behavioral dysfunction, or those who are bedfast and needing total care
- Are receiving hospice care / services
- Have end-stage renal disease
- Are under the age of 55 years old
- Have mental illness or mental retardation
- Communicate with non-oral communication devices, sign language, or who speak a language other than the dominant language of the facility

The survey team will look at other areas whether or not concerns have been identified. These areas include:
- Resident Funds – to find out whether the facility has enough surety bond for resident funds, and whether funds are turned over to resident after discharge, or whether funds are turned over to the legal estate of the resident after death of a resident(if your state has a regulation that is more stringent than the Federal regulation you go with the more stringent regulation)
- Infection Control – the surveyor will talk to the staff responsible for Infection Control. The surveyors will review infection control policies and procedures, and observe facility practices

- Record on Influenza Vaccine, and Pneumococcal vaccine – the surveyors will review the facility record to ensure that vaccines are administered to residents as required by the regulations during the flu season
- Quality Assurance Review – the surveyors will talk to the staff responsible for Quality Assurance. The surveyors will ask about incident and accidents record keeping and analysis by the facility. The surveyors will need to see evidence that the facility has an active incident accident prevention program and all incidents and accidents are reviewed, investigated, analyzed, and trended by the facility.
- Nursing Services
- Nurse staffing, sufficient staff to provide care for the residents

Other Major Areas of Focal Review and Information Gathering to Determine Compliance

- The surveyor(s) assigned will do a detailed Assessment of the environment of the facility to determine whether the facility is maintaining a safe and clean environment to enhance the residents' life, health, and safety. The surveyors will also observe and assess whether the environment portrays a homelike impression, or whether the environment looks too institutional.

- The surveyor(s) assigned will do a detailed Assessment of the Kitchen/Food Service Department's food storage, preparation, and service. The surveyor will score the kitchen for compliance with State regulations as well.

- The survey team will do detailed Resident Review – the surveyors will assess drug /medication therapies; quality of life issues including resident to resident interaction and staff to resident interaction; care concerns identified; dining observations; and closed record review.

- The surveyor(s) assigned will do a detailed Quality of Life Assessment – they will do individual resident interviews; a group resident interview; family interviews; and also observations of residents who are non-interviewable.

- Care Observations and Interviews are performed by surveyors who have the clinical knowledge and skills to evaluate and determine compliance. The surveyors will observe the residents and caregivers during care and treatment in different care settings, such as wound dressing change to make sure that clinical protocols are followed. They will also observe whether care plans are written and implemented by all staff to address the residents' conditions. Are care plans revised appropriately? Is resident given pain medication as ordered? It is important to note that during care and treatment observation, the surveyors will be observing to see if the staffs are maintaining the privacy of the residents, including the privacy of the body.

- The consultant pharmacy of the survey team will observe Medication Pass and Pharmacy Services - to determine medication pass error rate; the provision of pharmacy services by a licensed pharmacist; the facility's policies and procedures in place regarding the acquiring, receiving, dispensing of medication to residents; quarterly pharmacy committee meetings; psychotropic drugs; physicians' responses to facility's consultant pharmacist's recommendations.

- There will also be record review, to help determine the accuracy of the assessments of the residents. The surveyors will review the Minimum Data Set (MDS) for accuracy, for timeliness of assessments, etc. In addition to record review of residents currently in the facility, there will be closed record review as well.

- The surveyor(s) assigned will review the facility's Prevention of Abuse program. Everyone I am sure is aware of the importance of the prevention of abuse program in long term care. The surveyor assigned will make a determination whether the facility's policies and procedures have the required components as stated in the law, to protect the residents from abuse, neglect, involuntary seclusion, and misappropriation of their funds and property. The policies and procedures should address hiring practices including background check, regular training of staff, and supervision of employees, reporting requirements/protocol within the facility, investigating allegations of abuse and reporting requirements to the State survey agency and other agencies.

A standard survey lasts an average of five days depending on the size of the facility. During the survey period the survey team meets daily to share information amongst them. The team coordinator may meet with the administrator daily to report issues or concerns that they notice during the survey, but this meeting does not happen if there are no concerns to report.

I want to underscore here that regardless of the surveyors' tasks during the survey, please be mindful that the surveyors are always observing and watching – they are observing the environment, they are observing the residents, and they are observing staffs' interaction with residents. The facility must be resident-centered; the care provided for the residents must be resident-centered; and the survey also is resident-centered.

If sub-standard quality issues or concerns surface during the survey or if immediate jeopardy issues surface during the survey, the survey will last much longer, and this may lead to an extended survey.

Exit Conference

At the end of the survey, the survey team will conduct an exit conference with the facility's key personnel, or with the staff/personnel that the administrator invites to the exit conference. The team leader and the rest of the survey team will go through their survey findings, including potential deficiencies.

Form CMS-2567

Form CMS-2567 is the deficiency report compiled by the survey team of the facility's survey performance. CMS-2567 shows a listing of the deficiencies and F-Tags that the facility did not meet long term care regulatory requirement(s). This report is usually completed by the survey team in about ten days after the end of the survey.

Survey Protocol and Survey Process
Quality Indicator Survey

CMS implemented this computer assisted long term care survey process, the Quality Indicator Survey (QIS) to also determine if long term care facilities are in compliance with the Medicare and Medicaid conditions of participation. The objectives of this new form of computer assisted survey are as follows. The QIS survey will:

- Improve consistency and accuracy of quality of care and quality of life problem identification by using a more structured process;

- Enable timely and effective feedback on survey processes for surveyors and managers;

- Systematically review requirements and objectively investigate all triggered regulatory areas within current survey resources;

- Provide tools for continuous improvement;

- Enhance documentation by organizing survey findings through automation; and

- Focus survey resources on facilities (and areas within facilities) with the largest number of quality concerns.

Survey Protocol and Survey Process

The survey process for QIS format has been revised to enable automation of some parts of the process, and CMS continues to reinforce that the Federal Regulations and the Interpretive Guidelines remain unchanged. This survey utilizes the customized software on tablet personal computers (PC) to guide surveyors through their structured investigation.

1. **Pre-survey preparation usually called Offsite Survey Preparation**. The survey team coordinator or team leader and survey team will prepare for the QIS survey as they do for the Traditional Survey except for the automation portion. The offsite QIS preparation includes:
   - Review of the facility's prior deficiencies and plan of correction.
   - Review of the facility's current complaints and complaint surveys

- Talk to Ombudsman to find out if there are any complaints or concerns about the facility
- Identify areas of concerns
- Minimum Data Set (MDS) data for the facility are loaded offsite into the surveyors' tablet PCs (this is new with the QIS)

2. **Entrance Conference** – the team coordinator will meet with the Administrator and the Director of Nursing. (This may vary because the team coordinator decides who needs to be in entrance conference). The team coordinator will give the administrator a two page list of information/document needed by the survey team. The information/documents requested are listed in #4 through #7 below.

3. **The survey team members will do a concurrent initial brief tour of the facility to gain an impression of the facility.**

4. The administrator will need to provide the following information immediately at the end of the entrance conference.
- **An alphabetic resident census,** with room numbers/units. (Residents who are in the hospital or on therapeutic leave should be noted on the census).
- The **completed New Admission Information form**, which has a listing of all new admissions who were admitted 30 days before the start of the survey. This list will include Admission date, Date of Birth, Room Number/Unit
- The team leader will ask the administrator to post survey announcement signs in high-visibility areas such as the lobby.
- A copy of the facility's floor plan.
- A copy of the staffing schedules for licensed practical nurses and registered nurses during the survey period.

5. The administrator will provide the following information **within one hour after the end of the entrance conference**.
- A list of the key personnel in the facility
- The name of the president of the resident council, or an officer or active member of the council
- The schedule of meal times and the location of the dining room(s)
- Medication administration times
- Closed records of all those residents in the Admission Sample residents provided, who are discharged from the facility. The survey team will review these records throughout the survey.
- If the facility employs paid feeding assistants, the team leader will ask the administrator whether the paid feeding assistants' went through a State approved training program. Requirement is for feeding assistants to undergo a minimum of 8 hours of training in a program approved by the State.

- The team leader will also ask for names of the paid feeding assistants, and the names of residents who are receiving assistance from the paid feeding assistants.

6. The administrator will provide the following information/documents **within four hours after the end of the entrance conference.**
   - A list of residents who received the Preadmission Screening and Resident Review (PASRR) Level II services. The PASRR is a task usually done by the Social Worker for residents admitted. It may vary from facility to facility as to which discipline performs the PASRR.
   - A list of residents receiving dialysis care; the policies and procedures about care coordination with the dialysis facility, the plan of care for these residents, and contract/agreements with the dialysis facilities
   - If there are residents in the facility that are receiving home dialysis services the administrator will provide the names, room numbers and name of ESRD caregiver or technician.
   - The Influenza and Pneumococcal Immunization policy and procedures.
   - Any resident's rooms that require a variance such as room(s) that does not meet the required footage; room(s) with more than four residents; room(s) below ground level; room(s) with no window to the outside; and room(s) with no direct access to an exit corridor.
   - The name of the chair of the Quality Assurance Committee, names of committee members, and the frequency of meetings.
   - Information if any of experimental research done in the facility.
   - The name of the person responsible for the Prevention of Abuse Policies and Procedures, the Complaints and Grievance program in the facility.

7. The administrator will provide the following information/documents **within 24 Hours of the entrance conference**.
   - The completed Medicare/Medicaid Application (Form CMS-671)
   - The completed Resident Census and Conditions (Form CMS-672)
   - List of Medicare beneficiaries who requested a demand bill in the past six months of the survey
   - Information about the facility's emergency water source
   - Director of Nursing (DON) coverage – to ensure that full time coverage exists.

8. The team leader will also give the CASPER 3 report to the administrator.

Stage 1 Preliminary Investigation

There are three Stage 1 samples that are selected.

1. The first Stage 1 sample is the census sample. This census sample includes up to 40 randomly selected residents who are in the skilled nursing facility / nursing facility at the time of the survey. This sample is to help focus on quality of care and quality of life in the facility.

2. The second Stage 1 sample is the admission sample. The admission sample includes as many as 30 recently admitted residents; this includes admissions currently in the facility, and also discharged residents. This sample is to help focus on issues such as rehospitalization, death, or functional loss.

3. The third Stage 1 sample is the Minimum Data Set (MDS) data that is used to create the resident pool from which the Stage 1 samples are randomly selected, and to calculate the MDS-based Quality of Care and Quality of Life Indicators (QCLIs) for use in Stage 2.

Stage 1 Initial Review includes the following:

- Resident Interviews
- Family Interviews
- Staff Interviews
- Resident Observations
- Clinical Record Reviews

Mandatory tasks performed by the survey team for Stage 1 include:

- Interview of the president of the resident council
- Observation of the dining room(s)
- Observation of the kitchen
- Observation of the facility's Infection Control practices
- Observation of Medication Administration
- Review of the demand billing process
- Review of the Quality Assessment and Assurance Program

Completion of Stage 1 Review

After the completion of the stage 1 review, the surveyors using the onsite automation software will process the data collected through reviews and observations. Multiple observations would have been conducted to help identify care concerns or facility tasks. The survey team will determine which Quality of Care and Quality of Life Indicators (QCLIs) exceeded the national threshold of the long term care regulations. Those reviews or observations that exceed the national thresholds will trigger for further Stage 2 investigation and a more systematic, detailed, and organized care review. The survey team will identify all care areas and residents, which will be included in the Stage 2 sample.

Stage 2 Investigation

The survey team will perform an in depth investigation at the stage 2 level. The in-depth investigation involves conducting essential observations, and interviews, and also conducting relevant document review. The survey team will have in place the Critical Elements Pathway Forms for residents and care areas triggered, after the Stage 1 investigation. The Critical Elements Pathway Forms are then utilized to complete the Stage 2 reviews, interviews, and observations.

Below is listing of Critical Elements Pathways that are utilized for triggered residents for Stage 2 investigation:
- Activities; ADL and/or ROM Status
- Behavioral and Emotional Status
- Urinary Incontinence, Urinary Catheter, Urinary Tract Infection
- Communication and Sensory Problems
- Dental Status and Services
- Dialysis Treatment
- Hospitalization or Death
- Pain Recognition and Management
- Physical Restraint
- Pressure Ulcers
- Psychoactive Medications
- Rehabilitation and Community Discharge
- Ventilator-Dependent residents
- Review of Unnecessary Medication
- Preadmission Screening and Resident Review
- Hydration Status
- Tube Feeding Status

Below is a listing of Facility Tasks Pathway utilized for triggered care areas for Stage 2 in depth investigation.

- Admission, Transfer, and Discharge Review
- Environmental Observations
- Sufficient Nursing Staff Review
- Personal Funds Review
- QIS Extended Survey
- Abuse Prohibition Review

Completion of Stage 2 Investigation

At the conclusion of the in-depth care investigations and facility tasks that were triggered, the survey team will analyze the results to determine whether noncompliance with the Federal requirements exists. The computer software uses the same decision making process regarding scope and severity for noncompliance.

Exit Conference

At the end of the survey, the survey team will conduct an exit conference with the facility's key personnel, or with the staff/personnel that the administrator invites to the exit conference. The team leader and the rest of the survey team will go through their survey findings, including potential deficiencies.

Form CMS-2576

Form CMS-2567 is the deficiency report compiled by the survey team of the facility's survey performance. CMS-2567 shows a listing of the deficiencies and T-Tags that the facility did not meet long term care regulatory requirement(s). This report is usually completed by the survey team in about ten days after the end of the survey.

PART II

REGULATIONS AND F-TAGS

AND

MONITORING TOOLS

FOR

RESIDENT MEAL TIME & DINING EXPERIENCE

KITCHEN & FOOD SERVICE

How to Use the Monitoring Tools

The Monitoring Tools – Resident Meal Time & Dining Experience and Kitchen & Food Service are designed in an easy-to-read and easy-to-follow format. The monitoring tools reflect the current Federal Long Term Care Regulations and the Interpretive Guidelines. Staff can utilize these tools to help prepare for survey and to help with the task of ongoing monitoring for compliance. These tools are appropriate to help with all facilities whether the facility is a Traditional Survey facility or a Quality Indicator Survey facility.

Having interdisciplinary teams work together to observe resident meal times is helpful. The team can observe what happens when food carts are delivered to the floors or the units. They can observe whether the staffs make themselves available to serve the residents their meals, or whether the food stays unattended in the food service delivery cart for a while. They can also observe staffs interaction with the residents during meal time. If the facility has paid feeding assistants, are the paid feeding assistants working under the supervision of a Licensed Practical Nurse or a Registered Nurse? I need to state here that the facility will decide if they want to use teams to do the internal observation/monitoring or if they prefer individual staff members to do the observation or monitoring. It is the administrator' DON's or QA Director's choice if they use teams or individual staff persons.

The same goes for the kitchen. The facility can put their own internal teams together or have individuals to observe the kitchen and the food service staff for compliance. In addition to these monitoring tools the teams must also have available the State Dietary Manual, and other State requirements for food service. The staffs doing the internal monitoring must check freezer and refrigerators temperatures to ensure that the food is maintained at the proper temperature. All areas of the kitchen must be observed for compliance. Are leftover foods labeled and dated before they are placed in the refrigerator? Are food cooked to the proper temperature? Is the cold food kept at the proper temperature in the refrigerator? Is the kitchen floor clean? They can also check the dishwasher temperature for washing and rinsing cycles.

Facilities can work towards meeting CMS' expectation of consistent monitoring set for SNFs and NFs, by utilizing these tools in addition to other resources, for resident meal time, and for the kitchen and food service. These tools will help staff increase their comfort level of the regulations, while monitoring for compliance.

Listed in this section also are portions of the Federal Regulations and F-tags that reflect "Resident Meal Time and Dining Experience" and Federal Regulations and F-tags that reflect "Kitchen and Food Service".

The key for the monitoring tools are as follows:
Y = Yes
N = No
NA = Not Applicable

REGULATION F-TAGS

FOR

RESIDENT MEAL TIME AND DINING EXPERIENCE

Regulation: 42 CFR §483.15(a): Dignity; §483.15(h)(5): Adequate and comfortable lighting;
   §483.15(h)(6): Comfortable and safe temperatures;
   §483.15(h)(7): Comfortable sound levels; §483.20(a): Admissions Orders
   §483.25(a)(1)-(1V): A resident's abilities in ADL's do not diminish include Eating
   §483.25(A)(3): Resident unable to carry out ADL receive good nutrition, grooming.
   §483.35(d): Food; §483.35(d)(4): Substitutes offered similar nutritive value
   §483.35(e): Therapeutic Diets; §483.35(f): Frequency of meals
   §483.35(f): Frequency of meals; §483.35(h): Paid Feeding Assistants
   §483.70(g): Dining and Resident Activities;
   §483.75(f): Proficiency of Nurse Aides

The list below gives you a quick easy-to-read and easy-to-follow shortened format of the related F-tags for both the Traditional Survey and the Quality Indicator Survey (QIS).

F241 – The facility must promote care for resident in a manner to **enhance resident's dignity and self respect.**

F256 – The facility must provide **adequate and comfortable lighting in all areas.**

F257 – The facility must provide **comfortable and safe temperature levels.**

F258 – The facility must maintain **comfortable sound levels**

F271 – Admissions Orders – At the time resident is admitted, **physician order for immediate care, which includes diet.**

F310 – The resident's abilities in **activities of daily living (ADL) do not diminish unless circumstances of the individual clinical condition demonstrate that diminution was unavoidable; this includes Eating**

F312 – A resident who is unable to carry out activities of daily living receives the necessary services to maintain good nutrition, grooming, and personal and oral hygiene?

F364 – Food – The facility prepares food in manner that conserve nutritive value, flavor, and appearance; and that the food palatable, attractive, and served at proper temperature?

F366 – Substitutes - The food prepared as **substitute is of similar nutritive value to residents who refuse food served?**

F367 – Therapeutic Diets- the **resident to receive Therapeutic Diets** as prescribed by attending physician

F368 – Frequency of Meals – The facility to **provide three (3) meals a day at regular intervals with 14 hours between the substantial evening meal and the breakfast meal the following day. The facility must offer snacks at bedtime daily.**

F373 – Paid Feeding Assistants – If facility has paid feeding assistant, **did the paid feeding assistants go through a State-approved training course?**

F464 – Dining and Resident Activities – The facility must provide appropriate **one or more rooms designated for dining and activities; room must be well lighted, well ventilated, adequately furnished.**

F498 – Proficiency of Nurse Aides – Nurse Aides must show competency annually in skills and techniques to care for residents' needs.

RESIDENT MEAL TIME AND DINING EXPERIENCE MONITORING TOOL

Resident Medical Record # _____

F241 – Resident's Dignity and Self Respect

Regulation & Interpretive Guidelines	Compliance Y / N / NA	Comments
Is the resident well groomed?		
Does staff make resident's meal available to all residents at the table as soon as meal is delivered to the unit/floor?		
Does staff provide napkins and silverware (non-disposal) flatware to eat their meal?		
Does staff sit beside the resident while feeding the resident?		
Does staff interact and speak with resident while assisting resident with meal?		
Does staff address resident in respectful and courteous manner?		
Does staff allow resident to eat their meal at their own pace as opposed to rushing resident to finish meal?		
Does staff maintain a quiet dining room experience with little or no loud talking amongst staff members?		
Does the facility promote care for resident in a manner to enhance resident's dignity and self respect?		

F256 – Adequate lighting

Does the facility provide adequate lighting in common areas including the dining room(s)?		
Does the facility provide adequate lighting in residents' rooms?		

NOTES

F257 – Temperature levels

Does the facility routinely provide comfortable temperature level for residents?		
Does the facility provide temperature that is maintained between 71 – 81 degrees Fahrenheit range for good dining experience?		

F258 – Sound Levels

Does the facility maintain comfortable sound levels for residents and staff?		
Does staff have to raise their voices and compete with background noise?		
Does the resident have difficulty hearing what is being said due to background noise?		

F271 – Admission Orders

Does the resident have doctor's orders for his/her diet?		
Is the resident receiving the proper diet ordered by his/her doctor?		

F310 – A resident's abilities in activities of daily living relative to eating

Is the staff aware that the regulation states that the resident's abilities in activities of daily living (ADL) do not diminish unless circumstances of the individual clinical condition demonstrate that diminution was unavoidable?		
For resident requiring assistance, does the staff give resident the required assistance as stated in care plan?		
Does the resident need assistive device/utensils to eat meal?		
Does the resident need cueing or prompting to eat and is staff providing the required assistance?		

For resident requiring feeding, is resident being fed timely when the food is delivered to floor/unit?		
Is food served to resident within the required food temperature for both hot and cold food?		
Is all the staff available during meal time to ensure all residents receive their meal timely?		
Is the staff aware of risk factors that may affect the resident's eating abilities to chew and swallow?		
Is the staff aware that the resident's oral health may negatively affect the resident's eating abilities?		
Is the staff aware that a deficit in neurological and muscular status can negatively affect a resident from effectively moving food to eating utensils and to the mouth?		
How well does the staff know the wishes of the resident – does the staff know whether the resident likes to eat in his/her room or in the dining room?		
Does the staff know the resident's food likes and dislikes?		
Does the staff know whether the resident prefers to eat at different times as opposed to the scheduled meal times?		

F312 – Requirement for facility ensure that a resident who is unable to carry out activities of daily living receives the necessary services to maintain good nutrition, grooming, and personal and oral hygiene

Is the staff fully aware of the level of assistance needed by the resident?		
Does the staff demonstrate their awareness to provide the necessary services to maintain good nutrition, grooming, and oral hygiene, for those residents who cannot carry out activities of daily living?		
Is the staff aware that the services for oral hygiene include brushing the teeth, cleaning dentures, cleaning the mouth and tongue either by assisting the resident with a mouth wash or by manual cleaning with gauze sponge?		

NOTES

F364 – Food- the resident must receive and the facility must provide food that conserve nutritive value, flavor, and appearance; and that the food is palatable, attractive and served at the proper temperature

For resident who may require mechanical soft or puree diet, does the food look attractive, and is the food palatable, and does the food preserve the nutritive value?		
Does the resident food maintain the required food temperature?		
Does the resident meal routinely look attractive on the plate, and palatable?		

F366 – Substitutes – Food prepared and offered as substitutes of similar nutritive value to residents who refuse food served

When a resident refuses the food served, is the resident offered a substitute of similar nutritive value?		
Is the substitute consistent with the usual and ordinary food items provided by the facility?		
Does the staff anticipate substitutes based on the resident's food likes and dislikes compared to the menu items?		
Does the resident have to wait long periods for the substitute to be delivered to the resident?		
Does the substitute have similar nutritive value as the original menu item?		

F367 – Therapeutic Diets

Is the resident receiving therapeutic diet?		
Is the therapeutic diet prescribed by the resident's attending physician?		

F368 – Frequency of Meals

Does the facility provide at least three meals a day at regular intervals as comparable to that in the community for the residents?		
Is the interval between substantial evening meal and breakfast the following day about 14 hours or less?		
Does the facility offer snacks at bedtime daily?		
When snacks are routinely offered at bedtime, does the facility offer breakfast a little beyond 14 hours but not to exceed 16 hours between the substantial evening meal and breakfast the following day?		

F373 – Paid Feeding Assistants

Does the facility have paid feeding assistants on staff?		
Does the facility limit paid feeding assistants services only to residents who do not have complicated feeding problems?		
Does the paid feeding assistant demonstrate an awareness that he/she should not assist resident with complicated feeding problems?		

F464 – Dining and Resident Activities

Is the designated dining room well ventilated, with good air circulation?		
Are furnishings structurally sound and functional?		
Are chairs of appropriate and varying sizes meet the varying needs of the residents?		
Can wheelchairs fit under the dining room table?		
Is there sufficient space to accommodate all residents that want to eat in the dining room?		

F498 – Proficiency of Nurse Aide Program

As direct care givers, do certified nursing assistants demonstrate their proficiency and skills in taking care of the residents' needs as identified in resident assessments, and outlined in the care plan?		
Is the staff providing the activities of daily living services to meet the needs of the residents?		
In addition to meeting the feeding needs of the residents, does the staff provide adequate liquid at mealtime to meet residents' needs?		

NOTES

REGULATION F-TAGS

FOR

KITCHEN AND FOOD SERVICE

Regulation: 42 CFR §483.35(d): Food; **§483.35(i)(1):** Store, Prepare and Distribute Food; **§483.35(i)(3):** Dispose of Garbage and Refuse Properly; **§483.65(a):** Infection Control; **§483.70(c)(2):** Maintaining Essential Equipment **§483.70(h)(4):** Maintaining Effective Pest Control

Below are the F-tags for the above referenced regulations both for the Traditional Survey and the Quality Indicator Survey. (Remember the Regulation has not changed. "The F-tags remain the F-tags")

F364 – Food

F371 – Storing, Preparing, Distributing and Serving Food under Sanitary Condition

F372 – Properly Disposing of Garbage and Refuse

F441 – Infection Control (To focus on the section Relative to Food Service)

F456 – Maintaining Essential Patient Care Equipments and Mechanical Equipments

F469 – Maintaining Effective Pest Control

KITCHEN AND FOOD SERVICE
MONITORING TOOL

F364 – Food

Regulation & Interpretive Guideline	Compliance Y / N/ NA	Comments
Does the facility prepare food by methods to conserve the flavor, appearance and nutritive value of the food?		
Is the food palatable, attractive and prepared at the proper temperature?		

F371 – Store, Prepare, and Distribute Food

Does the facility procure food from approved and satisfactory sources?		
Is food stored properly under sanitary conditions?		
Is raw meat stored away from vegetable and other foods in the refrigerator?		
Is raw meat stored separately from cooked foods when stored in the refrigerator?		
Is staff aware of the required temperatures that foods must be cooked, maintained and stored in order to prevent food borne illness?		
Is staff aware that hot foods should leave the kitchen or steam table above 140° F		
Is staff aware that cold food should leave the kitchen at or below 41° F?		
Is staff aware that freezer temperatures should be 0° F or below?		
Is staff aware that refrigerator temperature should be maintained at 41° F or Below?		
Does the staff label and date leftover food stored in the refrigerator?		
Does the staff wash their hands prior to preparing, serving and distributing food?		
Is frozen food thawed in the refrigerator?		
Does the staff use sanitized thermometer to evaluate food temperatures?		

Are potentially hazardous foods kept at an internal temperature of 41° F or below in cold food storage unit, or at internal temperature of 140° F or above in hot food storage unit during display and service?		
Is leftover food heated to the appropriate temperatures?		
Does staff minimize hand contact with food?		
Does the food delivery system to residents' dining room and resident rooms protect the food from contamination?		
Are hand washing facilities convenient and properly equipped for dietary staff and dietary service use?		
Are cans and containers of food stored properly off the floor and on clean surfaces to prevent contamination?		
Are areas under storage shelves kept clean regularly?		
Is food transported in a way that protects against contamination?		
Is the food area free of pests?		
Is there any sign of rodent or insect infestation?		
Does the dishwashing procedure follow the 1993 Food Code, DHHS, FDA, PHS recommended temperatures?		
Does the dishwashing machine maintain 140° F for the wash cycle, and 180° F for the rinse cycle?		
For manual wash does the water temperature stay 170° F for 15 seconds?		
Does the 3 compartment sink use the sanitized solution per manufacturer recommendation?		

F372 – Dispose of Garbage and Refuse

Is garbage and refuse container in good condition?		
Is waste properly contained in dumpsters or compactors with lids covered?		
Is the garbage storage area maintained in good condition to prevent harborage and feeding of pests?		
Are garbage receptacles covered when being removed from the kitchen area to the dumpster?		

NOTES

F441 – Infection Control (Kitchen and Food Service)

Does the facility have a system to monitor and investigate causes of infection and manner of spread of infection?		
Does the facility program include risk assessment of occurrence of communicable disease for both residents and staff that is reviewed annually?		
Does the kitchen staff use gloves in accordance with aseptic principles?		
Does facility prohibit staff with open areas on their skin, signs of infection or other indication of illness, from handling food products?		

F456 – Maintenance of Essential Equipments in safe Operating Condition

Are the kitchen refrigerator and freezer in safe operating condition?		
Is the equipment maintained according to manufacturer recommendation?		

F469 – Maintain Effective Pest Control

Does the facility demonstrate effective pest control program?		
Is the facility free from rodents and pests?		

NOTES

PART III

ENFORCEMENT

BRIEF SYNOPSIS

PART III

ENFORCEMENT – Brief Synopsis of Enforcement

After an annual certification survey, or any Federal or State survey, the long term care facilities, including skilled nursing facilities (SNFs) and nursing facilities (NFs) will be required to submit an acceptable plan of correction within the required timeframe, which is 10 calendar days from receipt of the deficiency report Form CMS-2567, if deficiencies are cited during the survey. If there are no deficiencies cited or if the deficiency is Level A, that means the facility has a very successful survey, and no plan of correction is required. If however a facility incurs an immediate jeopardy (IJ) citation for their survey, this clearly is not a good outcome for the facility. A facility with an "IJ" will not be allowed to submit a plan of correction until *after* the facility removes the immediate jeopardy (see discussion on immediate jeopardy below).

Acceptable Plan of Correction – For detailed discussion on acceptable plan of correction, refer to Chapter 7 State Operations Manual §7304.4 (Revised with Effective Date of 09-10-10, and Implementation Date of 09-10-10)

Except in cases of past noncompliance, facilities having deficiencies (other than those at scope and severity level A) must submit an acceptable plan of correction. The requirement for a plan of correction can be found in 42 CFR 488.402(d) and §7400.2 and §7400.5.3, Appendix P.

I am highlighting below the requirements for an acceptable plan of correction. If the facility's plan meets these requirements there is a very good chance that the plan will be accepted and approved by the survey agency as "An Acceptable Plan of Correction".

Requirements:
- The plan of correction must address how corrective action will be accomplished by the facility staff for those residents found to have been affected by the deficient practice; *and*

- The plan of correction must address how the facility staff will identify other resident having the potential to be affected by the same deficient practice; *and*

- The plan of correction must address what measures the facility staff will put into place or what systemic changes will be made to ensure that the deficient practice will not recur; *and*

- The plan of correction must indicate how the facility staff plans to **monitor** their performance to make sure that solutions put in place are sustained; *and*

- The plan of correction must include dates when corrective action will be completed. The corrective action completion dates **must** be acceptable to the State.

If the plan of correction is unacceptable for any reason, the State will notify the facility in writing. If the plan of correction is acceptable, the State will notify the facility by phone, email, etc. Facilities should be cautioned that they are ultimately accountable for their own compliance, and that responsibility is not alleviated in cases where notification about the acceptability of their plan of correction is not made timely.

The **plan of correction** serves as the facility's allegation of compliance with regulation. Without it, CMS and/or the State have no basis on which to verify compliance. A plan of correction must be submitted within 10 calendar days from the date the facility receives its Form CMS-2567, Deficiency Report. If an acceptable plan of correction is not received by the survey agency within this timeframe the State will notify the facility that it is recommending to the Regional Office (RO) of the Centers for Medicare and Medicaid Services and/or the State Medicaid Agency that remedies be imposed.

Because "**immediate jeopardy**" is such a severe matter, it is the requirement by CMS and the State that, for most cases of immediate jeopardy, the facility must submit an **allegation of removal** of the immediate jeopardy. Facilities with "immediate jeopardy" violations have unfortunately demonstrated severe negative outcome(s) which puts the residents' health and safety in immediate jeopardy. There are situations when some facilities worsen the problem of putting health and safety of residents in immediate jeopardy with **substandard quality of care**. When immediate jeopardy is observed during the survey, surveyors will immediately inform the Administrator and Director of Nursing that their facility has an immediate jeopardy citation and the facility must take immediate steps to remove that citation. Immediate jeopardy in the "Deficiency Matrix or Grid" is any deficiency that is either a "J", or "K", or "L".

It is required that the allegation provided by the facility *for the removal of the **immediate jeopardy** include the date the immediate jeopardy was removed, and sufficient details demonstrating that the immediate jeopardy has been addressed.* Once the removal of the immediate jeopardy is verified, the surveying entity will provide the deficiency report Form CMS-2567, to the facility, including the noncompliance which constituted immediate jeopardy; and request that a plan of correction be submitted within 10 calendar days.

Listing of Remedies - Chapter 7 State Operations Manual §7400 (Revised with Effective date of 09-10-10, and Implementation Date of 09-10-10)

7400.3.1 – Available Enforcement remedies

In accordance with 42 CFR 488.406 below is the list of available remedies:

- Termination of the provider agreement;

- Temporary management;

- Denial of payment for all Medicare and/or Medicaid residents by CMS;

- Denial of payment for all new Medicare and/or Medicaid admissions;

- Civil Money penalties;

- State Monitoring;

- Transfer of residents;

- Transfer of residents with closure of facility;

- Directed plan of corrections;

- Directed in-service training ; and

- Alternative or additional State remedies approved by CMS.

§7400.5.1 address the factors that affect the selection of the appropriate remedy or remedies for a facility's noncompliance. The seriousness of the deficiency must first be assessed. The factors that determine which deficiency will be assessed include:

- No actual harm with a potential for minimal harm;

- No actual harm with a potential for more than minimal harm but not immediate jeopardy;

- Actual harm that is not immediate jeopardy; or

- Immediate jeopardy to resident health or safety.

And, whether the deficiencies:

- Are isolated;

- Constitute a pattern; or

- Are widespread.

See Deficiency Matrix and Remedies Next page

The Deficiency Matrix and Remedies

Immediate Jeopardy to Resident Health or Safety	Level J - PoC Remedies Cat. 3 is Required Cat. 1 is Optional Cat. 2 is optional	Level K - PoC Remedies Cat. 3 Required Cat. 1 Optional Cat. 2 Optional	Level L - PoC Remedies Cat. 3 Required Cat. 2 Optional Cat. 1 Optional
Actual harm that is not immediate	Level G – PoC Remedies Cat. 2 is Required* Cat.1 is Optional	Level H - PoC Remedies Cat. 2 Required* Cat. 1 Optional	Level I – PoC Remedies Cat. 2 Required* Cat. 1 Optional Optional: Temporary Mgmt.
No actual harm with potential for more than minimal harm that is not immediate jeopardy	Level D - PoC Remedies Cat. 1 Required* Cat. 2 Optional	Level E – PoC Remedies Cat. 1 Required* Cat. 2 Optional	Level F – PoC Remedies Cat. 2 Required* Cat. 1 Optional
No actual harm with potential for minimal harm	Level A – No PoC Not on CMS-2567	Level B	Level C
	Isolated	Pattern	Widespread

REMEDY CATEGORIES

Category 1	Category 2	Category 3
Directed Plan of Correction	Denial of Payment for New Admissions	Temp. Mgt.
State Monitoring, and/or	Denial of Payment for All Individuals imposed by CMS; and/or	Termination
Directed In-Service Training		Optional:
	Civil money penalties	Civil money penalties
	$50 - $3,000/day	$3,050-$10,000/day
		$1,000 - $10,000/ Instance
	$1,000 - $10,000/instance	

The State Survey Agency, or the Regional Office (RO), usually sends a letter with the survey results Form CMS-2567. The letter is addressed to the administrator of the facility, highlighting very important information and timelines the administrator needs to be aware of. The letter will include the date the survey was conducted, the timeline for the submission for the plan of correction if that is what is required, the requirements for the plan of correction, and which survey remedy is being imposed based on the severity of the deficiencies on the survey findings.

If a facility is in **substantial compliance**, and the survey finds isolated deficiencies with no actual harm and potential for only minimal harm, this is classified as a **(Form A) deficiency**, for which no plan of correction is required. The deficiency or deficiencies however should be corrected by the facility. The letter from the State survey agency will stipulate that a plan of correction is not required for the Form A deficiency report, but that the deficiency or deficiencies need to be corrected by the facility.

If another facility demonstrates **substantial compliance also**, but that facility's survey deficiencies **constitute a "pattern" or "widespread" findings** causing "no actual harm with the potential for minimal harm" to the residents, the State survey agency's letter or RO's letter whichever applies, will instruct the facility to submit a plan of correction to the State survey agency or RO within ten calendar days. This deficiency or deficiencies are level B and Level C. The plan of correction must be an acceptable plan of correction. Although this facility was in substantial compliance, a level B or level C requires that the facility submits a plan of correction. The benefit of level B and level C is that the surveying agency will not do a revisit to validate compliance, but the facility must comply with the plan of correction submitted.

If a third facility's survey resulted in the facility **not being in substantial compliance,** this is level D and above. The survey agency will do a revisit to the facility three months after submission of an acceptable plan of correction. If that facility still fails to maintain substantial compliance within three months after it has being found to be out of compliance, a Category 2 Remedy can be imposed, which may result in **Denial of payment for new admissions**. Other category 2 remedies include Denial of Payment for All Individuals (residents) in the facility, and civil money penalties. CMS and the State survey agencies have several options based on the severity of the deficiencies.

Civil money penalties, denial of payment for new admissions, and denial of payment for all residents in the facilities are remedies that speak to the conditions of participation in the Medicare and Medicaid programs. The ultimate goal is for facilities to provide resident-centered quality of care and quality of life for their residents, so when facilities do not meet that goal under the conditions of participation, CMS enforces the remedies.

If a facility is found to provide **substandard quality of care on three consecutive standard surveys**, **Denial of payment and State monitoring** may both be imposed. If however substandard quality of care is cited for the first time, and depending on the severity of the deficient practice, the survey team has an option to levy a category 1 remedy or category 2 remedy on the facility. Substandard quality of care is a deficient practice that results in "actual harm that is not immediate" and this deficient practice is usually a level G, or level H, or level I on the deficiency matrix.

Administrators must be aware of an additional remedy for immediate jeopardy. If an immediate jeopardy exists that jeopardize the health and safety of the resident and also constitute a substandard quality of care, the survey agency will notify the attending physician of the resident, as well as notify the State Board that is responsible for the licensing the facility's administrator. So administrators' names will be sent to their State Nursing Home Administrator Board.

Important information for facilities to note as well is that the Centers for Medicare and Medicaid Services or the State Medicaid Office may impose "Termination" of a facility's operations at any time depending on the severity of the substandard quality of care violation(s).

*If alternative remedies are imposed instead of, or in addition to termination, then this is required.

REFERENCES

Footnotes 1, 2, 3: State Operations manual Chapter 7 – Survey and Enforcement Process for Skilled Nursing Facilities and Nursing Facilities, (Rev. 09-10-10) page 11

State Operations Manual Appendix PP Guidance to Surveyors for Long Term Care Facilities rev. 1/7/11

State Operations Manual Chapter 7 – Survey and Enforcement Process for Skilled Nursing Facilities and Nuring Facilities (Rev. 09-10-10)

Deficiency Matrix- "Survey & Enforcement Process for Skilled Nursing Facilities and Nursing Facilities"

Printed in the United States
By Bookmasters